I0449816

Essential Oils
How To Make Your Own Essential Oil Perfume

Table of content

Introduction

There you are, in the department store once more, looking over the selection of perfumes that are on display. You recognize the names of singers, designers, movie starts, and every other person imaginable, but you don't know that you want to smell like the scent they have on display.

You flip over the boxes to take a look at what is on the back, and you find that there are countless words you can't pronounce, things you haven't ever heard of, and the description doesn't seem to fit you at all, so you are left wandering about, trying to find the perfume that is right for you.

But again and again you look, and again you are met with the same issue. Either you don't like the scent, you don't like the ingredients they put into the perfume, or you don't like the celebrity that is on the scent.

You don't want to support animal testing, whether it comes from the company directly or if it happens to be one of the parent companies... it doesn't matter to you. You want to know that no creature was harmed during the production of your perfume, and you want to wear the scent with pride knowing for a fact you are the one who best represents the scent.

"I can't find anything that fits what I want, and so many of the perfumes cost way more than what I want to spend on them anyway."

"I wish I could pick a scent that matches me and what I want, not a scent that has nothing to do with anything I am interested in."

"I want to show the world how I feel when I walk through a room. I want to leave with them an impression of my being there."

If you have ever felt any of these opinions or emotions, you are not alone. So many women out there want to make an impression with their perfume, and so many more don't want to use the chemicals that are in the standard scent.

This book is going to change all of that once and for all, ending your struggle. You are going to get not only what you want, but exactly what you need. Something as uniquely perfect as you are.

Chapter 1 – Getting Started

Of course when you prepare to start any kind of new hobby you are more than eager to just jump right on in, but I have to warn you, if you don't do it right, you are going to end up with perfume that doesn't smell good, doesn't smell for very long, or doesn't smell at all.

Perfume is a touchy substance, and you have to deal with it properly in order to get it to not only smell good while it is on you, but to also smell good long term. Nothing is worse than opening up your drawer to get your perfume out of it and find that your scent has long since turned sour.

That is why I am going to get you started on the right course. In this chapter, we are going to take a look at the things you need before you even begin, so when the time does come to put the liquid together, you will have everything you need handy.

The un-perishables: Gathering your standard supplies

Perfume making can cost you a bit of money to get started in, but thankfully, there are so many things you can reuse in this hobby once you are up and running, it isn't going to cost you much at all to keep it going.

The first thing you will need is a small glass bowl.

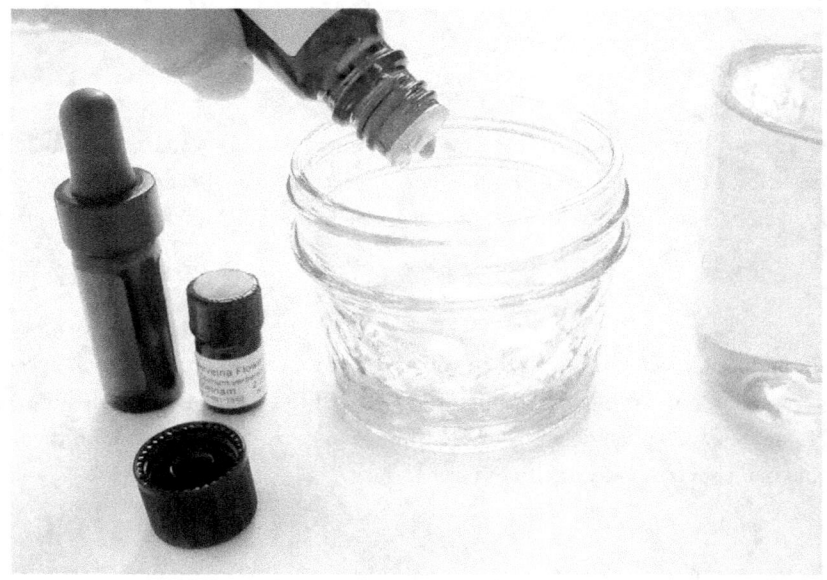

Of course you can use a glass you have on hand, but I like to keep my things separate, so I purchased and kept a small glass bowl in with my other perfume making items. It keeps it cleaner that way, as well as makes it a lot easier to find when you are ready to mix up some goods!

I recommend you also purchase a small measuring cup, an eye dropper, and a mixing needle

While you will use eye droppers more than a measuring cup, there are always things you will want on hand in case the event happens for you to want to use them. More often than not I find having a measuring cup on hand has saved me in a pinch, and if I ever don't need it, I just leave it in my box of supplies.

An eye dropper is the best way to measure how much of the oils you use in a mix, and I suggest you purchase a scientific grade eye dropper rather than a medicinal one. The scientific eye dropper is going to be smaller in the spout, and it will have a finer point to drip the oil out of.

This is going to make combining the oils a lot easier, especially when you are working with intricate recipes.

Of course, for the mixer, you can use anything you like, but I suggest you find a glass mixer to use if you are able. They are fragile, so you need to be careful when you are mixing your oils, but they are worth it.

I find wood or aluminum can react with certain oils, and you don't want to accidentally ruin a batch of perfume because you mixed it with the wrong material and ended up having a reaction in your cup! Glass is universally safe when it comes to plunging it into your oils, so have fun with it and make sure you are attentive as to where you put the mixer when you aren't using it.

Finally you will need containers to put your perfume in when it is ready.

I'm sure you are very familiar with spritz perfume, spray perfume, and roll on perfumes. No matter where you go to buy your perfume, you are bound to run into one or all three of these kinds of applicators.

No matter what your preference is, you are going to find just what you need either in a crafting store, or on Amazon dot com. Amazon has a huge source of perfume bottles, from the most basic roll on bottles to elaborate glass bottles that are pretty enough to be decorations all on their own.

Choose your favorite, or, better yet, mix and match to find the bottle of your choice, and you are going to have that perfect little touch to add to your perfect little mix. Just remember that any kind of applicator or bottle you choose to get needs to be taken care of, and glass is glass, so it can break really easily.

Be gently with it at all times, from pouring in the perfume initially to when you use it, and you will have perfume that lasts for ages to come.

Chapter 2 – The Ingredient List: Perishables

In the last chapter we looked at the things you will need to mix your perfume, but that is only the first half of the battle. If you want to make perfume, you are going to need the ingredients to make perfume out of.

Now, if you were to go into the store and flip over a jar of perfume, you are going to find all kinds of things listed in the ingredients that you can't pronounce. Perhaps you know what some of them are, but more than likely you won't have any idea. Not to mention even if you do know what the substances are, you don't want to have to try to track it down to put into your perfume.

No, you want something that is easy to blend, easy to come by, and gives you the results that you want. Thankfully, when you are into the natural way of life, you know that there are plenty of natural options you have to choose from to make your perfume.

The one thing I do want to point out, however, is that these items are perishable, which means they can get broken, they can get ruined, and they can expire. Just because you make a perfume that lasts for months, it doesn't mean the oil you have in your cupboard is going to last for the same amount of time if you don't use it.

You need to pay attention to the directions that are on the bottles of the ingredients you use, and make sure you follow those directions accordingly. The more care you put into the maintenance of the ingredients, the longer they are going to last you, and the more perfume you will be able to make.

So, let's get down to it, and discover what perishable items you are going to need to make your perfumes.

Essential oils

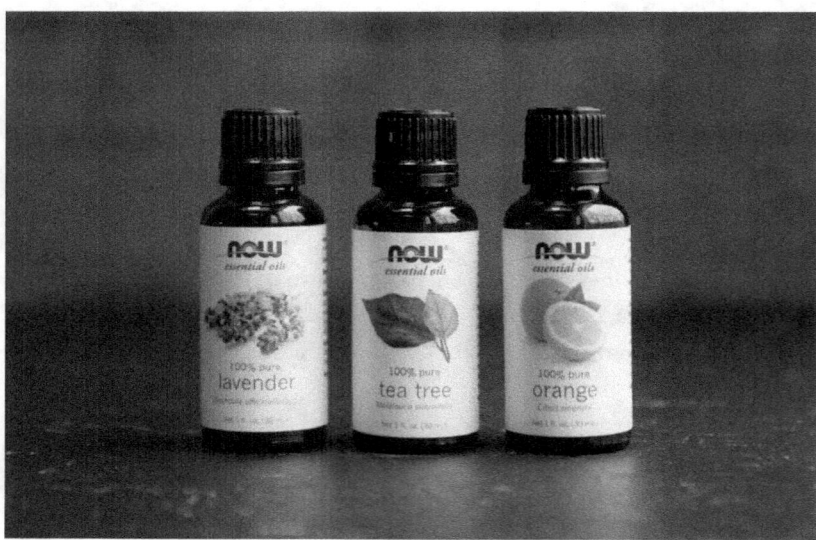

Obviously, you are going to need a selection of essential oils to choose from as you make your perfumes. More likely than not you have your box of oils as it is, but if you don't, don't worry.

In the chapters to come I am going to list specific oils to use in perfumes, and they are easily accessible on Amazon.

Remember that you can use the normal essential oils, or you can use the aromatherapy oils in your perfume. Both are natural, and you are going to get a lot more scent out of the aroma therapy grade oils.

Have fun with them and mix and match. Find out what you like, and go with that.

You will need a few drops of each kind of oil you use when you make perfume, so don't stress about finding a really big bottle. Even the smallest of bottles you find for sale on Amazon are going to have more than enough oils to let you make a few batches of perfume out of them.

Carrier oils

In addition to the essential oils, you are going to need a few carrier oils to blend into the perfume as well. I know it sounds strange, but the carrier oils act as a dilution to the oils, making them both smell great and keeping them from damaging your skin.

If you don't know which carrier oil is right for you, I suggest you use coconut. Simply search in a department store, or go online and you will easily find fractionated coconut oil.

This is exactly what you need as coconut oil is good for the skin, it is easy to come by as well as inexpensive, and it doesn't have a strong scent of its own so you don't have to worry about the carrier oil clashing with your specific scent.

You will also find avocado oil, almond oil, sweet almond oil, and other common carrier oils in any place you decide to look for them, so don't be afraid to try out what you like and what works for you.

Alcohol

Yes, you are going to need a good swig of alcohol to make your perfect perfume, and I'm not talking about tossing it back, but alcohol is essential if you want to make sure your perfume gets... and holds... that luxurious scent.

The key to making this work is simple: the higher the alcohol content, the better. Sure, you can use rubbing alcohol if that is all you have on hand, but if you are able to get your hands on some vodka, or better yet, everclear, you are going to find your perfume turns out so much better.

These are really the basic... but ever important rules of thumb that you shouldn't ever ignore if you want your perfume to turn out nicely. You will have to do your part in determining what is the best scent for you, as well as how much to use, but if you follow these ingredients for the guidelines, you are going to get perfumes that work in the long run.

Chapter 3 – Do This Not That: Common Mistakes and How To Avoid Them

No matter what your new hobby is, you are going to have a trial period in which you determine how it is going to work for you. There are going to be things that you take to right off, and there are going to be those ever embarrassing mistakes that you make.

But, mistakes are just what you need to take your skills from the bottom to the top, and in time, you are going to find that it is the mistakes you make that teach you the greatest lessons, and make you better able to know how to handle things later on.

So with that in mind, here are the most common mistakes first time mixers make, and what you can do to avoid them. You are going to have to work at it, and of course even with this list you are bound to make a few of your own, or even some of the same mistakes that I list here, but my point is you can pick yourself up and move on, and there's no real harm done in the long run.

Mistake number one: you skip or substitute ingredients that you shouldn't

Water is a very common item most people have on hand. It's clear, odorless, and easy to come by, so many people mistakenly feel that they can drop it into their perfumes to extend it, or to skip on one of the other ingredients.

As nice as it would be to be able to do this, I am sorry to inform you that you really can't substitute water for anything in the perfume, and I really recommend that you don't add it into the mix at all.

Water dilutes the perfume, which means it is going to take away the scent. It also evaporates quickly, which is another issue for scent loss. Water is also a different texture than the oil, and you will find the oil separates, and it is hard to mix it back together.

Bottom line is:

Avoid water in your perfume at all costs!

Mistake number two: you don't test as you go with the mixes

Tossing in a few drops of this and a couple drops of that sounds good in theory, but the result could be a disaster if you don't know exactly what you're getting at the end of the day.

To avoid this, simply test as you go, whether you use your stick to drop a drop on your arm or if you simply test it in the bottle itself. No matter how you do it, you need to make sure you are aware of how you mix smells before you dive in for the end result, or you may wish that you had.

Mistake number three: a little is good, a lot is better

This is a major mistake that many make when they are working with the aroma therapy grade oils. Sure, you can do this when you are working with the normal essential oils as well, but when you are using the aroma therapy oils, it is easy to get caught up in the delicious smells.

Make sure you are always thinking of things in miniscule amounts. Drips and drops are more than enough in most cases, and as I already said in the last section, you have got to test as you go, or you are going to end up with a disaster that you don't want to have to deal with.

Keep it on the modest side, and you will end up with a mix that is perfectly modest all around.

Mistake number four: you don't store your perfumes properly

I know there are a lot of different styles of perfume bottles on Amazon, and if you look at any other supplier, you are going to be bombarded with all kinds of different bottles to store your perfume in. I warn you to be careful, however, because if you don't store your perfume properly, it is likely to get ruined or lose its scent.

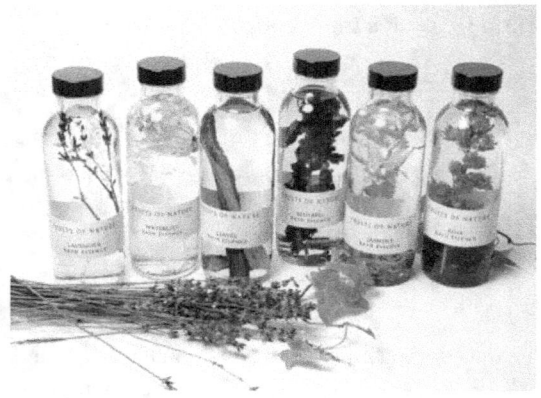

As a general rule of thumb, make sure you are using dark bottles. If the oils you use don't come in dark bottles, don't use them for your perfume, because they aren't the pure oils you are after.

True, pure essential oils are going to come in dark brown bottles. They may be small or on the larger side, but they are going to be definitely dark. And quality is something you can't compromise on no matter what you are doing.

Check to make sure your bottles are dark, whether you are using them for your perfumes, or if you are using the oils that come in these bottles. A little bit of precaution now is going to save you a lot of headache later on down the road.

Mistake number five: understand, and respect, the expiration date

The perfume you have on your night stand now may still smell great, even after a couple of years in the bottle, but that is a feature you aren't going to get when you use all natural perfumes.

Now, I am not saying that they are going to go bad in a matter of days, but you have to keep time in perspective when you are using them. If you are making them for the holidays, make sure you make them close to Christmas, or the time when you are going to be gifting them, and make sure you let your recipients know that they need to use them in a timely manner.

It's not a negative thing, but it is something to be aware of if you are going to make your own perfumes. Letting everyone know that they can be old is the best way to ensure everyone gets the best experience out of using them.

So don't be afraid to encourage the use of the oils in any way, you can always make smaller batches at a time, and enjoy the longer lasting scent that way!

Chapter 4 – Final Touch: Choosing The Right Scent For You

I wish when I was younger that someone would have told me then the art of finding my own perfume. I'm not saying that I couldn't find a perfume that I liked, I'm pointing out that the perfume that my friend would wear that smelled so good on her didn't have the same effect on me, and I had no idea why!

When it comes to perfume of any kind, your body is going to react to the oils differently, no matter what kind of oils you use, or how much you use. Your skin has its own oils, and as such it is going to make it a bit of a challenge to know exactly what it is going to smell like when it gets on you.

I recommend that you test a bit of it before you exhibit the final product, and that when you make your perfumes for your friends and family that you realize what smells one way on you may not have the same exact scent on another.

I find the best way to work around this is to make the scent as best as I can in the bottle. This means you are going to judge, mix, and match based on what you smell while it is in the mixing bottle, and not while it is on you.

If you are making yourself a perfume, then by all means test it on you to make sure you are happy with the scent, but if you are going to gift the scent, there is no shame in mixing the scent in the bottle and gifting it that way. Your recipient is going to be thrilled with it, and you don't have to worry that you customized it too much to suit your own preferences.

Keep in mind as well that there are oils you don't want to be putting on your skin, and even with a carrier oil it can be hard to know how much you can safely use when you apply it to your skin. I suggest you still avoid the hot oils, such as pepper, chili, or anything with a burn to it.

You can read up on all of the oils as you purchase them so you know which oils have that burn to them. Either way, start slow and go from there. There's nothing wrong with coming back to add more of a mix later on than putting in too much of it at first.

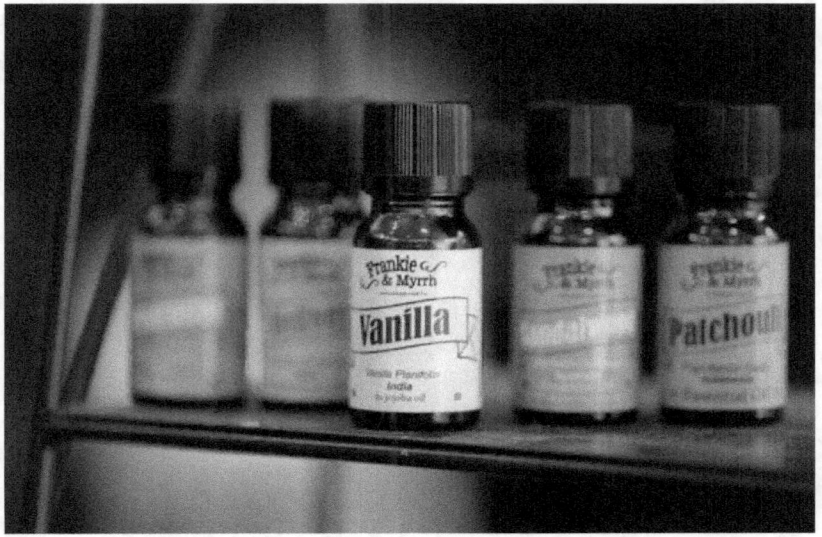

The more you are patient and practice with it, the better it is going to be for you in the long run.

So with that in mind, let's get down to it, and discover the top five recipes you can make for your all natural perfumes.

In addition to the basic blending that you are going to have in the recipes to come, I want you to practice the science behind it.

I know that sounds scary up front, but when you think about it, it's really easy.

As a general rule of thumb, and we know I love rules of thumb, you need to blend a floral scent, or a sweet scent of any kind, with something that is a little muskier. As a habit of life, try to mix and match the scents that are sweet with those that are low.

Think of it has notes. You want to have the overall scent as what comes through, such as the peppermint scent in the peppermint patty perfume you are going to find in the next chapter. But, peppermint isn't the only oil that you will be able to detect in the blend.

There will be other upper and lower notes that you will be able to smell, and you will find that they all come together to make the glorious blend that you have in your bottle when you are done. As you practice, you will get good at this, and in no time at all you will be able to pick and choose the blends that you want to make the perfumes you're thinking of.

This is when you will be able to make the perfumes as gifts, or when you will better be able to develop your own signature perfume.

No matter how you go about doing it, just make sure you have fun, and that you always love the results you make.

There is no failure, there's just the mistakes that turned into something great, and the mistakes that taught you how to do things a little differently the next time around.

Chapter 5 – To The Test: The Recipes

As I have already said, for each of these perfumes I recommend you test it out on your skin, and that you add a little at a time to make sure you get what you want for yourself.

But, each of the perfumes is going to use the same base, so I have included the recipe for the base of the perfume first. In each of the recipes, simply add in the essential oils, and you will get the perfume you are after!

No matter what you use for your perfume, your bottle, or in your base, remember that you do need to shake well before use. Shake gently, and make sure it is mixed before you apply.

The Base

3 tablespoons carrier oil of your choice

1 tablespoon alcohol of your choice. (If you are using rubbing alcohol, use 1.5 tablespoons)

Combine in a separate dish, then place in the bottle of your choice. Make sure you leave an inch or so at the top to add in your oils, and fill the rest of the jar with carrier oils when finished.

Please take note that these recipes are for ½ ounce bottles, and you will have several bottle's worth of perfume when you are finished.

The Fairy Princess

5 drops rose oil

4 drops patchouli

4 drops lavender oil

3 drops orange oil

The Peppermint Patty

5 drops peppermint oil

3 drops lemon oil

2 drops wintergreen

Sunshine and Picnics

5 drops lemon oil

4 drops hibiscus oil

3 drops lemongrass oil

Day at the Beach

6 drops hibiscus oil

5 drops lilac oil

5 drops lavender oil

5 drops sandalwood oil

Happy Life

6 drops lemon oil

6 drops lime oil

5 drops sweet orange

5 drops vanilla oil

Of course, these are just the basic measurements for these perfumes. I like this blend for each of these perfumes myself, but you are going to have the freedom to play around with them and discover what it is you like the best.

There's no wrong way to do it, you just need to mix and match until you are happy with what you have. Explore your collection and the different mixes I have here, and you will be amazed with what kind of blends you can come up with!

The results are endless, you just need a bit of imagination and some time to practice, and you can have any kind of blend, any time you want.

So what are you waiting for?

You have perfume to make.

Conclusion

There you have it, everything you need to know to get you started in making your own perfumes, and exactly what you need to know to change the way you wear perfume forever.

There are so many more factors that come into what you do besides the act itself, and when you don't know what goes into something before it hits the shelves, you are setting yourself up for disaster. Of course the companies like to keep their secrets under lock and key, but there are times when that doesn't work for you.

I hope this book was able to change all of that for you, and that you are now able to see that you really can make your own perfume, and you can control exactly what goes into it. You are in complete control over the ingredients, the scent, and the final product, and only you are able to make a scent that is as one of a kind as you are.

When you buy scent on the shelves of the store, you are choosing one bottle among many, meaning that you have to end up with the same signature that so many others have, and so many others use. You don't want that. You don't want to be just like everyone else, you want to be you, and you want to do it your way.

This book is going to change all of that, giving you the opportunity to make your own perfume your way, no matter what you want it to be. I know you have so many ideas bouncing around in your head, and with a little bit of direction, you can take those ideas and put them down into the bottle.

This book is going to open the door for you, giving you what you need to get into freedom. You will be able to dream it, make it, and own it, no matter what it is you want to do. This book is going to be your guide into the wild world of perfume, and once you enter in, there is no turning back.

You are going to be set no matter what holiday is coming up, no matter how many times you want to change up your own look, or how many times you want to shake things up and make them your own. This book is going to show you everything you need to know to get you out of the department store and into your kitchen, mixing it up to be just the way you want it.

You deserve to be spoiled, and perfume is by far the best way to do that. Don't ever settle for what anyone else is doing. Shoot for the best of the best, and you are going to have it.

So what are you waiting for? The door is open.

www.ingramcontent.com/pod-product-compliance
Lightning Source LLC
Chambersburg PA
CBHW061951280526
45787CB00004B/1819